DIARRHEA

DOCTOR'S ADVICE ON DIARRHEA

DR. J. SIMON

Contents

INTRODUCTION

Diarrhea is a common digestive illness characterized by frequent, loose, and watery bowel movements. There are multiple possible causes, and it is often a symptom rather than a singular illness. Diarrhea comes in two flavors: the short-lived acute diarrhea and the long-lived chronic diarrhea.

Causes of diarrhea:

Diseases caused by bacteria, viruses, or parasites can result in infectious diarrhea. Common pathogens include salmonella, norovirus, and Escherichia coli (E. coli).

Consuming contaminated or rotten food can result in food poisoning and other gastrointestinal distress, including diarrhea.

Medication: Certain medications, such as antibiotics, may cause diarrhea as a side effect and disturb the delicate balance of intestinal flora.

Food Intolerances and Allergies: Diarrhea may be caused by intolerances to specific foods, such as lactose or gluten, or by allergic reactions to those foods.

IBDs, or inflammatory bowel diseases, encompass ailments such as ulcerative colitis and Crohn's disease. Prolonged diarrhea may result from the inflammation of the digestive tract caused by these illnesses.

Malabsorption Syndromes: Disorders like pancreatic insufficiency or celiac disease that impair the body's capacity to absorb nutrients can cause chronic diarrhea.

Irritable Bowel Syndrome (IBS): IBS is characterized by recurrent episodes of diarrhea as well as bloating, stomach pain, and irregular bowel movements.

Stress and Anxiety: Emotional factors like stress and anxiety can contribute to diarrhea. Gastrointestinal symptoms are influenced by the connection between the brain and the stomach.

Symptoms of diarrhea include:

> - Frequent, loose, and watery stools
> - cramps and aches in the stomach
> - the urgent need to use the restroom
> - nausea and vomiting (in some cases)

Administration and Therapy:

Hydration: Especially if you have diarrhea, drink a lot of water to replace lost fluids and electrolytes from frequent bowel movements.

Dietary modifications: It can be helpful to follow a bland diet that avoids greasy or spicy foods and includes easily digested foods like toast, bananas, rice, and applesauce.

Medication: Over-the-counter antidiarrheal medications like loperamide (Imodium) can be taken to reduce the frequency of bowel movements.

Handling Underlying Causes: The treatment plan is dictated by the underlying cause. Antibiotics can be used to treat bacterial infections, and specific management methods are required for conditions like IBD and IBS.

Seeking Medical Attention: You should consult a doctor as soon as possible if you have severe or persistent diarrhea, especially if you are dehydrated, have a fever, or have blood in your stool.

Acute diarrhea typically goes away on its own, but severe or persistent episodes may indicate an underlying medical condition that needs to be properly diagnosed and treated. Always seek the advice of a qualified medical professional for specific advice and care.

CHAPTER ONE

Categories and Causes

Diarrhea can be divided into a number of groups according to its symptoms, underlying causes, and duration. Some common types of diarrhea and the causes of them are listed below:

1. acute diarrhea:

Causes: Acute diarrhea is often caused by illnesses like bacterial, viral, or parasitic diseases. Common pathogens include Shigella, Escherichia coli (E. coli), rotavirus, norovirus, and salmonella. Food poisoning and tainted water are frequent causes of illness.

2. Extended Diarrhea:

Causes: Chronic diarrhea is defined as diarrhea that persists for more than four weeks. Possible causes include Crohn's disease, ulcerative colitis, recurrent infections, certain medications, irritable bowel syndrome (IBS), and celiac disease.

3. Travel-related diarrhea:

Causes: Traveler's diarrhea is frequently brought on by consuming contaminated food or water while in unhygienic locations. pathogens such as E that cause bacteria. Coli are usually the culprits.

4. Inflammatory cholera:

Causes: Infectious diarrhea results in inflammation of the intestinal lining. The causes include bacterial, viral, or parasitic infections;

autoimmune diseases of the gastrointestinal tract; and inflammatory bowel disease (IBD) (also known as ulcerative colitis or Crohn's disease).

5. Osmotic diarrhea:

Causes: When the solute content of the intestine is higher than normal, water enters the colon and causes osmotic diarrhea. Among the causes are malabsorption syndromes, including lactose intolerance and celiac disease.

6. Secret diarrhea:

Causes: Secretory diarrhea is caused by increased fluid secretion into the intestines. Among the causes are infections, certain medications, and abnormalities in hormones.

7. Medication-Induced Diarrhea:

Causes: A variety of medications, such as cancer treatments, some antacids that contain magnesium, and antibiotics, can cause diarrhea by upsetting the normal balance of gut flora.

8. Differentiated Diarrhea:

Causes: The organic cause of functional diarrhea is unknown. Diseases such as IBS frequently cause changes in bowel habits without any sign of anatomical or biochemical abnormalities.

9. diarrheal discharge:

Causes: One sign of exudative diarrhea is the presence of blood and pus in the stool. Specific infections, inflammatory bowel disorders, and general infections can all cause exudative diarrhea.

10. Misinterpreted diarrhea

Causes: Malabsorptive diarrhea arises when the intestines are unable to properly absorb nutrients. Among the causes are pancreatic insufficiency, small bowel syndrome, and celiac disease.

Understanding the type of diarrhea and its underlying cause is essential for the proper diagnosis and treatment of the condition. A doctor's evaluation is usually necessary for cases of chronic or severe diarrhea in order to identify the exact cause and provide treatment, although some cases of acute diarrhea may resolve on their own. For a precise diagnosis and customized care, always consult a medical professional.

Diarrhea can show up as a range of signs and symptoms, depending on the underlying cause and severity of the illness. Typical signs and symptoms of diarrhea include:

Consistent, Unsteady, and Damp Poop:

Diarrhea is characterized by increased frequency of bowel movements, often with loose and watery stools.

Abdominal Pain and Cramps:

Many people with diarrhea experience abdominal pain, cramping, or discomfort. These symptoms have a range of intensities.

Urinary Movement Requirement:

Having a bowel movement may seem urgent, and those who have diarrhea may find it difficult to schedule or avoid them.

nauseated and vomiting:

Nausea and vomiting are common side effects of diarrhea, especially in cases of viral or inflammatory diarrhea.

An increase in temperature:

Fever may occur in conjunction with diarrheal infections. Elevated body temperature is a common response to diseases caused by bacteria, viruses, or parasites.

Dehydration:

Diarrhea-related fluid loss can result in dehydration. Weariness, dark urine, dry lips, and increased thirst are some signs of dehydration.

Sometimes mucus or blood in the stool indicates that a person has diarrhea. This could indicate underlying inflammation or damage to the gastrointestinal tract.

Weight Loss:

Severe or persistent diarrhea can cause weight loss due to the depletion of nutrients, electrolytes, and fluids.

Inadequacy and Weariness:

Weakness and exhaustion can be made worse by persistent or severe diarrhea, which is often associated with dehydration and nutritional depletion.

Bloating and stomach acid:

Bloating and increased gas production can occur along with diarrhea, especially when malabsorption or altered gut flora are involved.

Despite being a common symptom, diarrhea can be caused by a wide range of conditions, including infections, inflammatory bowel diseases, food intolerances, medications, and stress. The severity and duration of symptoms can vary, and severe or persistent diarrhea may require medical attention.

In certain cases, additional symptoms like joint pain, skin rash, or neurological symptoms may show up depending on the underlying cause of the diarrhea. When symptoms like fever, dehydration, prolonged abdominal pain, or blood in the stool are present along with diarrhea, it is best to get medical attention right away to ensure the right diagnosis and course of treatment.

Recognizing Diarrhea

A comprehensive review of the patient's medical history, a physical examination, and any additional testing required are used to diagnose diarrhea. The goals are to identify the underlying cause of the diarrhea and create an effective treatment plan.

Background Information on Health:

The medical professional will take a complete medical history and inquire about the frequency, duration, and onset of the diarrhea as well as any concomitant symptoms such as fever, nausea, or abdominal pain.

Dietary and lifestyle history:

Information regarding the individual's diet, recent travel, interactions with potential sources of infection, and any recent changes to their medication schedule or lifestyle will all be considered.

Physical Evaluation:

There may be a physical examination to assess vital signs, abdominal pain, and symptoms of dehydration. The medical expert may also look for additional physical symptoms that could provide information about the underlying cause.

Looking at the stool:

Stool samples can be collected for laboratory analysis to determine the presence of bacteria, viruses, or parasites. This test helps determine whether diarrhea is being caused by an infection.

Blood Tests:

Blood tests may be recommended to look for signs of infection, inflammation, or other abnormalities. A higher white blood cell count and inflammatory markers may indicate an underlying disease.

Colonoscopy or endoscopy:

In cases of severe or persistent diarrhea, a colonoscopy or endoscopy may be recommended to visually inspect the gastrointestinal tract. This treatment can identify inflammatory bowel disorders, polyps, and other anatomical anomalies.

Imaging Studies:

Two imaging modalities that can be used to evaluate the structure of the intestines and identify any abnormalities or obstructions are CT scans and abdominal X-rays.

Examining the Breath:

Hydrogen breath tests may be used to check for malabsorption issues such as lactose intolerance or bacterial overgrowth in the small intestine.

On rare occasions, an endoscopy or colonoscopy may involve an intestinal tissue biopsy. This can help with the diagnosis of inflammatory bowel disease and celiac disease, among other conditions.

Evaluation of Substance Use History:

The patient's medication history must be carefully reviewed in order to identify any medications that may be causing diarrhea as a side effect.

Evaluation of Prolonged Illnesses:

For persistent diarrhea, one may consider functional abnormalities, inflammatory bowel disease (IBD), and irritable bowel syndrome (IBS). Specific diagnosis criteria are used to determine the differences between these disorders.

The patient's symptoms, medical history, and clinical presentation will all be taken into consideration when developing the diagnosis plan. To get a proper diagnosis and treatment plan, people with severe or persistent diarrhea should see a doctor. Self-diagnosis and self-treatment may not solve the underlying issue, but getting help as soon as you can will help ensure proper care and avoid complications.

How diarrhea is treated depends on the underlying cause as well as the severity of the symptoms. Often, acute diarrhea resolves on its own without the need for additional medical attention. However, in cases that are severe or persistent, or when diarrhea is associated with other illnesses, targeted treatment approaches may be necessary. The following are common remedies for diarrhea:

consuming lots of water

It's critical to maintain adequate hydration, especially if you have diarrhea because fluid loss can lead to dehydration. Rehydration solutions, oral rehydration salts, and increased fluid intake are essential for replacing lost fluids and electrolytes.

Nutritional Modifications:

It is recommended to eat a bland diet and avoid foods that might aggravate diarrhea. Use the BRAT diet (bananas, rice, applesauce, and toast) to provide easily digested foods and reduce symptoms.

Substances:

Operamide (Imodium), an over-the-counter antidiarrheal medication, can help reduce the frequency of bowel movements. These medications should be used cautiously and under a doctor's supervision as they might not be suitable in all circumstances, especially if there is an underlying infection.

Managing Underlying Infections:

If the diarrhea is being caused by a bacterial, viral, or parasitic infection, antimicrobial medications may be advised. The course of treatment is determined by the specific infection discovered through laboratory testing.

Probiotics:

Probiotics are beneficial bacteria that may help improve gastrointestinal health and balance the gut flora. They might be useful in cases of antibiotic-induced diarrhea or infectious diarrhea.

Keeping Foods That Trigger:

People with food sensitivities or intolerances must avoid trigger foods that cause diarrhoea. Common triggers include dairy products, high-fat foods, and certain artificial sweeteners.

Managing Chronic Illnesses:

If diarrhea is associated with chronic illnesses such as irritable bowel syndrome, inflammatory bowel disease (IBD), or malabsorption disorders, the focus of treatment will be on treating the underlying condition. This may involve medication, dietary modifications, and lifestyle adjustments.

Anti-inflammatory medications:

Medications that reduce inflammation include corticosteroids and immunosuppressive drugs, which may be administered to treat the symptoms of inflammatory bowel diseases (IBD).

Modifications to Lifestyle:

Reducing stress, exercising frequently, and adhering to a healthy diet can all help to strengthen the digestive system and lessen the likelihood of recurrent episodes of diarrhea.

Receiving Medical Assistance:

If someone has severe or persistent diarrhea, they should seek medical attention as soon as possible, particularly if they also have other symptoms like fever, dehydration, or blood in their stool. This is necessary for an accurate diagnosis and appropriate treatment.

It's crucial to keep in mind that drug self-treatment, particularly with antibiotics, may not be appropriate in the absence of a proper diagnosis and medical guidance. The use of antibiotics can occasionally exacerbate an illness or lead to antibiotic resistance. Therefore, it is advisable to consult a healthcare provider for customized treatment depending on the specific cause of diarrhea.

dietary aspects

In order to manage diarrhea and promote healing, dietary factors are crucial. By altering the diet to include better-digestible and well-tolerated foods, symptoms can be lessened and the digestive tract can be prevented from becoming more irritated. The dietary recommendations listed below can be used to treat diarrhea:

BRAT Diet:

The BRAT diet is an acronym that stands for toast, applesauce, rice, and bananas. These foods are low in fiber, bland, and easy to digest. They can give you energy and aid in firming up stools without making your digestive system feel worse.

See-through Fluids:

Drink plenty of clear liquids, such as water, clear broths, and electrolyte solutions, to stay properly hydrated. To replenish fluids lost due to diarrhea and avoid dehydration, it is essential to stay hydrated.

Rich in Electrolytes Foods:

Eat foods high in potassium and sodium, which are rich in electrolytes. This covers rice, potatoes, bananas, and soups. In order to restore electrolyte balance, electrolyte solutions or oral rehydration solutions may also be helpful.

Steer clear of dairy products:

Dairy products should be temporarily avoided as they could be difficult to digest when experiencing diarrhea. Diarrhea can be a symptom of lactose intolerance, and avoiding dairy products can help reduce symptoms.

Low-Fiber Foods:

Eat fewer high-fiber foods because they can be more difficult to digest and worsen diarrhea.

White rice, refined grains, and thoroughly cooked, skinless vegetables are examples of foods low in fiber.

Trim Proteins:

Pick lean protein sources like tofu, skinless chicken, and fish. When compared to fatty or highly seasoned meats, these proteins are easier to digest.

Avert Greasy and Spicy Foods:

Eat less oily and spicy food because these can aggravate your digestive system. Choose foods that are simple and mildly seasoned to reduce irritability.

Small, Frequent Meals:

Eat smaller, more frequent meals throughout the day as opposed to one big meal. This can lessen the burden on the gastrointestinal tract and facilitate digestion.

Limit alcohol and caffeine:

Both alcohol and caffeine may aggravate the digestive tract and lead to dehydration. Limit or stay away from these drugs until your symptoms go better.

CHAPTER TWO

Fruits and Vegetables Cooked:

Select tender fruits and vegetables that have not been peeled; they are easier on the stomach. Easy-to-digest foods include cooked carrots, bananas, and applesauce.

Don't Use Sugar Replacements:

Some sugar-free products include sugar substitutes like sorbitol and mannitol, which can worsen diarrhea by acting as a laxative. Don't use these additives; always read labels.

Foods High in Probiotics:

Include foods high in probiotics, like yogurt with live cultures, in your diet. Probiotics have the potential to help the gut's beneficial bacterial balance be restored.

It's crucial to remember that food suggestions can change depending on the individual's unique situation and the underlying cause of diarrhea. A registered dietitian or other medical professional may offer specific advice in certain situations. It is advisable to seek medical attention for a proper diagnosis and treatment plan if the diarrhea is severe or continues.

Modifications to Lifestyle

In addition to dietary modifications, lifestyle changes can help control and prevent diarrhea. These modifications are made with the intention of enhancing digestive health in general and reducing variables that could aggravate symptoms. The following lifestyle recommendations are for people who have diarrhea:

Retain Hydration:

Regaining lost fluids from diarrhea requires drinking enough water. To avoid becoming dehydrated, consume lots of water, clear broths, and electrolyte solutions.

Solutions for Oral Rehydration:

To preserve hydration and restore electrolytes, think about taking oral rehydration solutions (ORS). When diarrhea is moderate to severe, these remedies are very helpful.

Avert Alcohol and Caffeine:

Both alcohol and caffeine can cause dehydration. Limit or stay away from alcohol- and caffeine-containing beverages until symptoms subside.

Relaxation and Rest:

Make sure you get enough sleep so your body can heal. Prioritizing rest and getting enough sleep is crucial because stress and exhaustion can affect digestive system performance.

Regular Exercise:

Regular moderate exercise can help support digestive health in general. However, during episodes of diarrhea, intense or vigorous exercise may need to be modified.

Maintain good hand hygiene to stop the transmission of illnesses that can lead to diarrhea. Before preparing or eating food, especially after using the restroom, thoroughly wash your hands with soap and water.

Manage Your Tension:

Diarrhea is one of the gastrointestinal symptoms that can be exacerbated by stress. To control your stress levels, try practicing mindfulness, meditation, deep breathing exercises, or yoga.

Steer clear of trigger foods:

Recognize and stay away from foods that can cause or exacerbate diarrhea. Foods that are spicy, high in fat, dairy products (if lactose intolerant), and some artificial sweeteners are common triggers.

Modest Dietary Adjustments:

To give the digestive system time to adjust, make dietary adjustments gradually. Digestion-related discomfort may be exacerbated by sudden dietary changes.

Review of Medication:

Consult a healthcare provider to go over your medication regimen and find any that might be causing diarrhea. Medication schedule modifications might be required with medical advice.

Frequent Health Examinations:

Keep an eye on your general health by scheduling routine checkups and screenings. Speak with a healthcare professional about any gastrointestinal symptoms that are ongoing or recurrent.

Precautions for Travel:

When visiting areas with varying levels of hygiene, exercise caution. Steer clear of raw or undercooked foods that could expose you to a risk of foodborne illness, as well as untreated water.

Speak with Medical Experts:

For severe or persistent cases of diarrhea, consult a healthcare provider. A prompt medical evaluation can assist in determining the root cause and recommend the best course of action.

It's crucial to remember that changes in lifestyle may be necessary depending on the underlying cause of diarrhea as well as the particular condition of the person. Seeking immediate medical attention is advised for a thorough evaluation and appropriate management if symptoms worsen or persist, or if dehydration is a concern.

Diarrhea in Particular Groups

People of all ages can get diarrhea, but some populations may be more susceptible to certain causes or complications related to the illness.

Regarding diarrhea in particular populations, keep the following in mind:

Young Children and Infants:

Infants and early children frequently have diarrhea, which is frequently brought on by infections, teething, or dietary changes. It is advised to breastfeed in order to supply vital nutrients and antibodies. To stop dehydration, oral rehydration solutions (ORS) might be suggested.

Senior Citizens:

Dehydration may be more common in older adults because of changes in the digestive system and a decrease in fluid reserves that come with age. Diarrhea may also be caused by medications that are frequently prescribed to senior citizens. It's important to stay hydrated and to keep an eye out for symptoms of dehydration.

Expectant Mothers:

Pregnancy-related diarrhea may result from infections, dietary modifications, or hormonal changes. A pregnant woman should drink plenty of water and speak with her doctor about the best course of action, taking into account any possible effects on the developing fetus as well as the mother.

Those with impaired immune systems:

Severe or protracted diarrhea may be more common in people with weakened immune systems, such as those with HIV/AIDS or receiving immunosuppressive treatments. In immunocompromised populations, infections that would normally cause mild diarrhea can have more serious consequences.

Travelers:

Traveler's diarrhea can strike people who are visiting places with varying levels of sanitation. Diarrhea can result from consuming tainted food or water. Visitors are urged to maintain the safety of their food and water, and they may think about taking preventative measures like immunizations or prophylactic medications.

People with Long-Term Illnesses:

Diarrhea can be recurrent or chronic in people with long-term conditions like celiac disease, irritable bowel syndrome, or inflammatory bowel disease (IBD). It's critical to manage the underlying illness, and dietary changes might be necessary.

People who have dietary intolerances or allergies:

Food allergies or intolerances, such as gluten sensitivity or lactose intolerance, can cause diarrhea. Identifying and steering clear of trigger foods is essential for symptom management.

Sportsmen:

Diarrhea brought on by exercise can be exacerbated by intense physical activity, particularly in endurance sports. Changes in blood flow to the intestines and dehydration might be factors. In addition to paying attention to proper hydration, athletes should think about making dietary adjustments both prior to and during exercise.

People in Institutional Environments:

People who live in long-term care facilities, hospitals, or nursing homes may be more vulnerable to infectious diarrhea outbreaks. In these cases, strict infection control measures and symptom monitoring are necessary.

Those undergoing intestinal surgery:

Patients who have had gastrointestinal surgery may experience diarrhea, especially if their intestines have been cut shorter or if their digestive systems are malfunctioning. Medical supervision and dietary modifications might be required.

It is important to take into account the unique factors that may contribute to or affect diarrhea for each specific group. Seeking proper medical advice and care is essential, particularly for vulnerable populations where complications or dehydration may pose a greater risk. Depending on a patient's health status, underlying conditions, and other relevant factors, healthcare professionals can modify interventions.

Issues and Prolonged Consequences

While most cases of diarrhea go away on their own or with appropriate treatment, persistent or severe cases can cause issues and potentially have long-term effects. Some concerns and problems associated with chronic or severe diarrhea include the following:

Dehydration:

One of the main effects of diarrhea is dehydration. Diarrhea can lead to electrolyte and fluid losses, which can result in dehydration. Particularly in vulnerable populations like young children, the elderly, or those with weakened immune systems, severe dehydration can be fatal.

The electrolyte disparity

Diarrhea may cause an imbalance in electrolytes, including sodium, potassium, and chloride. Electrolyte imbalances can have serious consequences, including irregular heartbeats and muscle weakness.

Lack of Nutrients:

Prolonged diarrhea may lead to inadequate dietary absorption and insufficiency of essential vitamins and minerals. This could affect overall nutritional status and lead to fatigue, weakness, and other health issues.

Weight Loss:

Because of the loss of nutrients, fluids, and electrolytes, chronic diarrhea can cause significant weight loss. Unintentional weight loss can have an effect on overall health and wellness.

Inflammatory or chronic diarrhea can cause damage to the gastrointestinal tract and lead to conditions like irritable bowel syndrome (IBS) or inflammatory bowel disease (IBD). These conditions may lead to long-term gastrointestinal issues and their effects.

Impact on Growth and Development (in Children):

Recurrent or chronic diarrhea may have an effect on a child's development and growth. Frequently falling ill and not getting enough nutrients can disrupt regular growth cycles.

Immunity deficit:

Prolonged or severe diarrhea may lower immunity, making people more susceptible to illness. Those with illnesses that impair their immune systems should pay particular attention to this.

Impact on the Mind:

Constant diarrhea can cause tension, anxiety, or depression, among other psychological effects. Managing chronic symptoms can be emotionally draining and negatively affect an individual's overall quality of life.

underlying medical conditions:

Extended diarrhea may be a sign of underlying medical conditions like inflammatory bowel disease (IBD), celiac disease, or recurrent infections. To guarantee long-term management, these fundamental problems need to be resolved.

Increased Risk of Colorectal Cancer (Under Some Circumstances):

With time, people with certain chronic inflammatory colon disorders, like ulcerative colitis, may have an increased risk of colorectal cancer. Appropriate medical management and routine monitoring are essential in these circumstances.

You should see a doctor if your diarrhea is severe or persistent, particularly if you are experiencing other concerning symptoms like weight loss, dehydration, blood in your stool, or other symptoms. A healthcare professional can conduct a thorough evaluation, identify the underlying cause, and offer an appropriate treatment plan to prevent issues and address long-term consequences.

Methods of Prevention

Preventing diarrhea requires lowering the risk of infection, promoting good hygiene practices, and making lifestyle choices that promote overall digestive health. Here are some strategies to avoid diarrhea:

Hand Hygiene:

Wash your hands well with soap and water after using the restroom, before eating, and after handling raw food. Keeping your hands clean aids in preventing the spread of diseases that can cause diarrhea.

Food Safety:

When handling and preparing food, exercise caution. Keep perishables in the refrigerator as soon as possible, cook meats thoroughly, and avoid contaminating raw and cooked food.

Safe Water Practices:

Sip safe, clean water. Avoid drinking untreated or contaminated water, especially when in unsanitary locations. Use treated or bottled water to drink; avoid eating ice that has been made from raw water.

Personal hygiene:

Maintaining personal hygiene reduces the risk of acquiring infections. If someone close to you has diarrhea, avoid them and do not share towels or cutlery with them.

Immunizations:

Ensure that your immunizations are current, especially if you are traveling to an area where certain infections, such as cholera or rotavirus, are prevalent. Consult with medical professionals to determine the right vaccination schedule.

Appropriate Food Storage:

Proper storage of food is necessary to prevent bacterial growth. Eat leftovers within a reasonable period of time and store them in the refrigerator as soon as possible. Food that seems to have gone bad ought to be thrown away.

Avoid consuming raw or undercooked food:

Meats, seafood, and eggs should never be eaten raw or undercooked because they could contain parasites or pathogenic bacteria that cause diarrhoea.

Avoid contaminated surfaces at all costs:

It is advisable to exercise caution when handling surfaces in public areas, especially in areas where there is a high risk of contamination. Hand sanitizer or washing should be done after handling surfaces in shared areas.

CHAPTER THREE

Probiotics:

Consider incorporating probiotic-rich foods or supplements into your diet. Probiotics may help maintain the right balance of gut microorganisms and improve digestive health.

Avoid using antibiotics excessively:

Antibiotics should only be taken as prescribed by medical professionals and should be used sparingly. Overuse or misuse of antibiotics can lead to an imbalance of gut bacteria, which is the cause of antibiotic-associated diarrhea.

Understanding and Awareness:

Remain informed about the causes of diarrhea and preventative measures. In particular, practice good hygiene in public settings and teach others the same.

Advice From Travelers Concerning Diarrhea:

When visiting areas where traveler's diarrhea is more likely, take extra precautions, such as avoiding strcct food, drinking bottlcd watcr, and being mindful of food safety.

Maintain a Healthful Lifestyle:

Adopt a healthy lifestyle that includes regular exercise, eating a balanced diet, and reducing stress. Maintaining a healthy lifestyle can help to improve digestive health overall.

By incorporating these preventive methods into their daily routines and maintaining good hygiene, people can reduce their risk of contracting illnesses that result in diarrhea. It is essential to tailor preventative measures to specific circumstances, such as travel destinations, age groups, and individual health requirements.

Diarrhea invoyeurs

Traveler's diarrhea is a common gastrointestinal illness that affects visitors to locations with differing standards of cleanliness, particularly those in developing countries. It is often caused by consuming or drinking food contaminated with bacteria, viruses, or parasites. The primary symptoms of traveler's diarrhea are as follows:

Bacterial infections: Salmonella, Shigella, Campylobacter, and Escherichia coli (E. coli) are common bacterial pathogens associated with traveler's diarrhea.

Infections caused by viruses: Rotavirus and norovirus are two viruses that can cause diarrhea, especially in contaminated or crowded environments.

Particularly in locations with inadequate water treatment, parasitic infections like Giardia lamblia and Cryptosporidium may be the cause of traveler's diarrhea.

Warning signs:

- ➢ diarrhea accompanied by puddles
- ➢ abdominal cramps
- ➢ emesis
- ➢ spitting up
- ➢ elevated temperature
- ➢ Headache

Preventive measures:

To be safe, only sip bottled or filtered water. Avoid using ice that has been created with raw water, and exercise caution while handling drinks that have ice in them.

Safe Food Practices:

Eat hot, thoroughly prepared food.

Avoid eating raw or undercooked shellfish, eggs, and meats.

Select peeled fruits and avoid raw vegetables and salads.

Hand Hygiene:

Wash your hands thoroughly with soap and water before and after using the bathroom.

Use hand sanitizer in the absence of soap and water.

Avoid eating street food:

Even if food on the street is frequently more appealing, there could be a higher risk of infection. Choose food from reputable suppliers.

Immunizations:

Consult medical professionals to determine the recommended vaccinations prior to traveling to regions where there is an increased risk of catching certain infections, such as cholera or typhoid fever.

Probiotics:

Consider taking probiotics before and throughout your trip to help maintain a healthy balance of intestinal bacteria.

Avoid polluted regions at all costs:

It is advisable to use caution when handling surfaces in public areas, especially in areas where there is a high risk of contamination.

Counseling:

Rehydration: Drink a lot of liquids, especially oral rehydration solutions, to prevent dehydration.

Antimicrobial Drugs:

Antibiotics are sometimes prescribed by doctors to treat bacterial infections that result in traveler's diarrhea. It is not recommended to self-treat with antibiotics without a proper diagnosis, though.

Reduction of Symptoms:

Over-the-counter medications, such as loperamide, can help alleviate the symptoms of diarrhea. However, if you have blood in your stool or a fever, you shouldn't use them.

Unwind:

Give your body time to heal and rest.

When to Seek Medical Assistance

The diarrhea lasts for more than a few days.

Lightheadedness, black urine, dry mouth, and extreme thirst are some of the severe symptoms of dehydration.

Either the feces contains blood or the fever is high.

It's imperative to consult medical professionals for personalized advice based on travel destinations, individual health conditions, and the likelihood of traveler's diarrhea.

CONCLUSION

In conclusion, diarrhea is a common gastrointestinal illness characterized by frequent, loose, or watery bowel movements. It could be caused by a variety of factors, such as underlying medical conditions, medication side effects, dietary choices, and infections. When treated appropriately, acute diarrhea usually goes away on its own, but severe or recurring cases can lead to dehydration, nutritional deficits, and electrolyte imbalances.

By leading a healthy lifestyle, cleaning your hands often, and ensuring the safety of your food and drink, diarrhea can be avoided. "Traveler's diarrhea" is a specific kind of diarrhea that is associated with traveling to places with poor sanitation; it can be prevented by taking the appropriate precautions, such as drinking clean water, eating hygienic food, routinely washing your hands, and getting the required vaccinations.

Diarrhea can be treated by combining dietary modifications with enough fluids and, if necessary, treating underlying causes. Lifestyle changes, such consistent exercise and stress management, can enhance general gut health.

Individuals who have severe or persistent diarrhea should seek medical attention as soon as possible, particularly if they are exhibiting other concerning symptoms. A healthcare practitioner may do a thorough evaluation, identify the underlying cause, and provide an appropriate treatment strategy to ease symptoms and prevent issues.

In general, when people are informed about the causes, preventative measures, and appropriate treatment procedures for diarrhea, they can take proactive steps to maintain gastrointestinal health and well-being.

THE END